TABLE OF CONTENTS

Introduction:

Welcome to "Beyond the Surface: Exploring Plastic Surgery for Body and Mind." In this book, we embark on a journey through the fascinating world of plastic surgery, where science, art, and the human spirit intersect. Plastic surgery has come a long way since its ancient origins, evolving into a multifaceted field that encompasses cosmetic enhancements, reconstructive procedures, and transformative surgeries that go beyond physical appearance.

At its core, plastic surgery is not just about changing one's appearance; it can be a catalyst for profound psychological and emotional transformations. As we delve into the various aspects of this complex discipline, we will explore the reasons people seek plastic surgery, the psychological impact of these procedures, and the ethical considerations that surround them.

This book aims to provide readers with a comprehensive and balanced understanding of plastic surgery, empowering them to make informed decisions, whether they are considering a procedure themselves or seeking knowledge about this dynamic field. Through in-depth exploration, we will unveil the history of plastic surgery, its diverse range of procedures, and the innovative techniques shaping its future.

We will also address the essential relationship between surgeons and patients, emphasizing the significance of trust, communication, and empathy in the journey of transformation. Beyond the operating room, we will investigate the psychological impact of plastic surgery, uncovering its potential to boost self-esteem and enhance overall well-being.

Yet, as we venture into this world of transformation, we must not overlook the ethical considerations and cultural implications of plastic surgery. We will delve into the societal pressures surrounding beauty standards, the influence of media, and the critical importance of embracing natural beauty and self-acceptance.

Moreover, we will shed light on the altruistic side of plastic surgery, exploring its significant role in reconstructive procedures and humanitarian efforts, where skilled surgeons bring hope and healing to those in need.

In the pages ahead, we hope to inspire a deeper appreciation for the artistry and science of plastic surgery. By fostering a nuanced understanding of its possibilities and limitations, we encourage readers to celebrate individuality, embrace natural beauty, and make informed choices that align with their own desires and values.

As we embark on this journey together, let us explore the transformative power of plastic surgery, not merely on the surface but within the realms of the human spirit, where empowerment, self-discovery, and compassion converge. Let us embark on this voyage of discovery with open hearts and open minds, guided by the belief that each individual's story and journey are unique and worthy of celebration.

Let us journey "Beyond the Surface."

Chapter 1: Overview of Plastic Surgery

Do's and don'ts

The decision to undergo plastic surgery is a significant one, and it is essential to approach the process with care and consideration. To help ensure a positive experience and satisfactory outcomes, here are some important do's and don'ts of plastic surgery:

Do's:

1. Do Your Research: Thoroughly research the procedure you are considering and the qualifications of the plastic surgeon. Look for board-certified surgeons with expertise and experience in the specific procedure you desire.

2. Do Seek Multiple Consultations: Consult with multiple plastic surgeons to gain different perspectives, understand the

potential risks and benefits, and make an informed decision.

3. Do Have Realistic Expectations: Understand that plastic surgery can enhance your appearance, but it may not completely change your life or solve all personal issues. Have realistic expectations about the potential results.

4. Do Disclose Your Medical History: Be open and honest about your medical history, including any medications, allergies, or past surgeries. This information is crucial for the surgeon to assess your candidacy and plan the procedure safely.

5. Do Follow Pre-Operative Instructions: Adhere to the pre-operative guidelines provided by your surgeon. This may include avoiding certain medications, alcohol, and smoking before surgery.

6. Do Arrange Post-Operative Care: Plan for adequate post-operative care and support during your recovery period. Follow your

surgeon's instructions for wound care, medication, and activity restrictions.

7. Do Attend Follow-Up Appointments: Attend all post-operative follow-up appointments with your surgeon to monitor your healing progress and address any concerns.

8. Do Maintain a Healthy Lifestyle: Leading a healthy lifestyle with regular exercise and a balanced diet can contribute to optimal healing and overall well-being.

Don'ts:

1. Don't Make Hasty Decisions: Take your time to consider the decision carefully. Avoid rushing into surgery without fully understanding the procedure and its potential consequences.

2. Don't Choose Based on Price Alone: Quality and safety should be prioritized over cost. Be cautious of offers that seem too good

to be true, as the quality of care may be compromised.

3. Don't Disregard Potential Risks: Understand and accept the potential risks and complications associated with the procedure. A thorough discussion with your surgeon will help you make an informed choice.

4. Don't Expect Perfection: While plastic surgery can achieve significant improvements, no procedure can guarantee perfection. Embrace your individuality and understand that natural variations are part of being human.

5. Don't Hide Information from Your Surgeon: Be honest and transparent with your surgeon about your expectations, desires, and any concerns you may have.

6. Don't Use Unrealistic Expectations from Photos: Avoid basing your expectations solely on before-and-after photos of other patients. Each person's anatomy and results are unique.

7. Don't Ignore Your Gut Feeling: If you feel uncomfortable or uncertain about the surgeon or the procedure, don't proceed. Trust your instincts and seek a second opinion if needed.

By following these do's and don'ts, you can approach plastic surgery with confidence and make decisions that are best for your well-being and aesthetic goals. Remember that open communication, informed choices, and realistic expectations are key to a successful and satisfying plastic surgery experience.

Post operative care

Post-operative care is a critical aspect of the plastic surgery journey, as it directly impacts the healing process and the final results. Proper post-operative care helps minimize complications, reduce discomfort, and optimize the overall recovery experience. Here are some general guidelines for post-operative care after plastic surgery:

1. Follow Surgeon's Instructions: Adhere strictly to the post-operative instructions provided by your plastic surgeon. These instructions may include wound care, medications, activity restrictions, and follow-up appointment schedules.

2. Take Prescribed Medications: Take all prescribed medications as directed, including pain relievers, antibiotics, and any other medications to aid healing and manage discomfort.

3. Manage Wound Care: Keep the surgical incision sites clean and dry as instructed by your surgeon. Follow any dressing change protocols and avoid soaking the incisions in water until cleared by your surgeon.

4. Avoid Strenuous Activities: During the initial recovery period, avoid any strenuous activities or heavy lifting as advised by your

surgeon. Allow your body to heal without putting undue stress on the operated area.

5. Wear Compression Garments (if applicable): If your surgeon recommends compression garments, wear them as instructed to minimize swelling and support the healing process.

6. Elevate the Operated Area: Elevate the operated area, if possible, to reduce swelling. For example, if you had facial surgery, use extra pillows to keep your head elevated while sleeping.

7. Maintain a Healthy Diet: Consume a nutritious diet that supports healing and helps the body recover. Stay hydrated and avoid foods that may interfere with medications or the healing process.

8. Avoid Smoking and Alcohol: Refrain from smoking and limit alcohol consumption, as these can impair the healing process and increase the risk of complications.

9. Attend Follow-Up Appointments: Attend all scheduled follow-up appointments with your surgeon. These visits allow the surgeon to monitor your progress, address any concerns, and provide further guidance.

10. Be Patient and Allow Healing Time: Remember that healing is a gradual process, and results may take time to fully develop. Avoid comparing your progress to others and focus on your individual recovery journey.

11. Reach Out to Your Surgeon: If you have any questions or concerns during the recovery period, do not hesitate to contact your plastic surgeon. They are there to support you and address any post-operative issues.

Remember that post-operative care is as important as the surgery itself. By following your surgeon's instructions diligently and taking care of yourself during the recovery period, you can promote a smooth and successful healing process, allowing you to enjoy the full benefits of your plastic surgery results.

Chapter 2: The History of Plastic Surgery

The history of plastic surgery is a rich tapestry that spans thousands of years, encompassing remarkable advancements and cultural influences. From ancient civilizations to the modern era, this branch of medical science has undergone significant transformations. Let's take a fascinating journey through time to explore the milestones and key moments in the history of plastic surgery:

Ancient Beginnings:
The origins of plastic surgery can be traced back to ancient civilizations, where rudimentary techniques were used for reconstructive and cosmetic purposes. In India, around 600 BCE, the practice of rhinoplasty was documented, as surgeons

attempted to reconstruct noses that had been amputated as a form of punishment.

In ancient Egypt, medical texts dating back to 3000 BCE mentioned techniques for repairing facial injuries. The Egyptians were also skilled in basic surgical procedures, such as wound closure and the treatment of abscesses.

Indian Influence and Innovations:
Throughout the centuries, India emerged as a significant hub for plastic surgery advancements. Sushruta, an ancient Indian physician often referred to as the "father of surgery," documented a vast array of surgical procedures, including innovative techniques for reconstructing the nose and ears.

Middle Ages and Renaissance:
During the Middle Ages, knowledge of plastic surgery waned in Europe, but it continued to thrive in other regions. The Arab world made significant contributions to the field, preserving ancient medical texts and advancing surgical techniques.

The Renaissance marked a revival of medical knowledge in Europe, and plastic surgery gradually reemerged. Italian surgeon Gaspare Tagliacozzi made notable contributions to reconstructive surgery in the 16th century, particularly in the realm of nasal reconstruction.

World Wars and Reconstructive Surgery: The First and Second World Wars had a profound impact on the development of plastic surgery. The surge in facial injuries and disfigurements during the wars prompted significant advancements in reconstructive techniques.

Innovations like the "tubed pedicle" and "free flap" procedures allowed for complex tissue grafting and reconstruction, enabling surgeons to restore form and function to injured soldiers and civilians alike.

Cosmetic Surgery Boom: In the mid-20th century, plastic surgery witnessed a surge in cosmetic procedures driven by advancements in anesthesia and surgical techniques. Procedures such as facelifts, breast augmentations, and liposuction became more common.

Modern Era and Technological Advancements:
The latter half of the 20th century saw exponential growth in plastic surgery with the advent of new technologies and materials. Microsurgery, endoscopy, and laser technology revolutionized the field, allowing for more precise and minimally invasive procedures.

Today, plastic surgery continues to evolve with ongoing research, technological innovations, and a greater emphasis on patient safety and ethical considerations. The field encompasses an array of specialties, including aesthetic surgery, reconstructive surgery, craniofacial surgery, and hand surgery, among others.

The history of plastic surgery is a testament to the human spirit's capacity for innovation and compassion. From its humble beginnings in ancient times to the cutting-edge techniques of the modern era, plastic surgery has transformed lives, restored confidence, and contributed to medical advancements.

As we move forward, the history of plastic surgery serves as a reminder of the discipline's enduring quest to blend science, art, and humanity, impacting lives beyond the surface and enriching the tapestry of human experience.

Chapter 3: The Different Types of Plastic Surgery

Plastic surgery encompasses a diverse range of procedures aimed at enhancing appearance, restoring function, and improving overall well-being. Let's explore some of the different types of plastic surgery:

1. Cosmetic or Aesthetic Surgery:
Cosmetic surgery focuses on improving the appearance of specific body parts or features. Some common cosmetic procedures include:

   a. Breast Augmentation: Enhancing breast size and shape through implants or fat transfer.
   b. Rhinoplasty: Reshaping the nose to improve its size and proportion.
   c. Liposuction: Removing excess fat from specific areas of the body.
   d. Facelift: Reducing signs of aging by tightening facial skin and muscles.

e. Tummy Tuck (Abdominoplasty):
Removing excess skin and fat from the
abdomen to create a more toned appearance.

2. Reconstructive Surgery:
Reconstructive surgery aims to restore the
function and appearance of body parts
affected by congenital defects, injuries, or
medical conditions. Some common
reconstructive procedures include:

a. Cleft Lip and Palate Repair: Correcting
congenital defects of the lip and/or palate.
b. Breast Reconstruction: Restoring the
breast shape and contour after mastectomy.
c. Burn Reconstruction: Restoring function
and appearance after severe burns.
d. Hand Surgery: Treating injuries,
deformities, and conditions affecting the
hands.

3. Craniofacial Surgery:
Craniofacial surgery involves addressing
congenital or acquired deformities of the
skull and facial bones. This type of surgery is

often performed on children with conditions like craniosynostosis or cleft lip and palate.

4. Microsurgery:

Microsurgery involves intricate procedures using specialized microscopes and instruments to repair or reconstruct small blood vessels, nerves, and tissues. It is commonly used in reconstructive surgeries like tissue transplantation and replantation of severed body parts.

5. Burn Surgery:

Burn surgery is dedicated to treating burn injuries, including skin grafting and other procedures to restore function and improve appearance.

6. Hand Surgery:

Hand surgery focuses on treating conditions and injuries affecting the hand, wrist, and fingers. This can include repairing fractures, treating carpal tunnel syndrome, and reconstructing hand deformities.

7. Gender-Affirming Surgery:
Gender-affirming surgery, also known as gender confirmation surgery or sex reassignment surgery, involves procedures to align an individual's physical appearance with their gender identity. This can include procedures like facial feminization surgery or genital reconstruction.

8. Body Contouring:
Body contouring procedures are designed to reshape and sculpt the body after significant weight loss, often following bariatric surgery or through natural means. These procedures may include body lifts, thigh lifts, and arm lifts.

Each type of plastic surgery serves unique purposes and addresses specific needs. Whether reconstructive or cosmetic, plastic surgery plays a vital role in improving the quality of life for individuals and enhancing their sense of self-confidence and well-being. It is essential to consult with a qualified plastic surgeon to discuss individual goals, expectations, and potential outcomes before undergoing any procedure.

Chapter 4: The Psychological Aspect of Plastic Surgery

The psychological aspect of plastic surgery is a crucial and multifaceted component of the decision-making process for both patients and surgeons. Plastic surgery involves not only physical transformation but also emotional and psychological considerations that can profoundly impact patients' well-being and self-perception. Let's delve into the various psychological aspects of plastic surgery:

1. Motivations for Plastic Surgery:
Understanding the motivations behind
seeking plastic surgery is essential. Some
individuals seek cosmetic procedures to
enhance their self-confidence and body
image, addressing specific insecurities they
may have about their appearance. Others may
desire cosmetic changes to align their
physical appearance with their internal sense
of self, particularly in gender-affirming
surgery. On the other hand, reconstructive
surgery patients may be seeking functional
and aesthetic improvements after injuries,
trauma, or congenital conditions.

2. Body Dysmorphic Disorder (BDD):
Body Dysmorphic Disorder is a
psychological condition characterized by an
obsessive preoccupation with perceived flaws
in one's appearance. Patients with BDD may
seek plastic surgery as a way to alleviate
distress, but surgery may not resolve their
underlying psychological issues. Ethical
plastic surgeons carefully screen patients to
identify those with BDD and refer them for

psychological evaluation and treatment when necessary.

3. Realistic Expectations:
Establishing realistic expectations is vital for both patients and surgeons. Plastic surgeons should communicate openly with their patients about the potential outcomes of the procedures, addressing any misconceptions or unrealistic expectations. Patients must understand that plastic surgery can enhance their appearance, but it may not solve all of life's problems or eliminate all insecurities.

4. Pre-Surgical Counseling:
Pre-surgical counseling plays a crucial role in the psychological aspect of plastic surgery. It allows patients to discuss their motivations, concerns, and expectations with the surgeon. During counseling, patients can gain a clearer understanding of the procedures, the recovery process, and potential risks and benefits. This process helps ensure that patients are emotionally prepared for surgery.

5. Post-Surgical Adjustment:

The post-surgical period can be emotionally challenging for some patients. It is essential to provide post-operative support and follow-up care to address any emotional concerns or complications that may arise during the recovery process. Patients may experience a range of emotions, including anxiety, depression, or dissatisfaction with results, and having support systems in place is crucial.

6. Impact on Self-Esteem:
Positive outcomes from plastic surgery can have a significant impact on patients' self-esteem and body image. Feeling more confident and comfortable in their appearance can lead to improved social interactions, increased self-assurance, and enhanced overall well-being.

7. Ethical Considerations:
Plastic surgeons have an ethical responsibility to prioritize the well-being and mental health of their patients. This includes the obligation to turn away patients who may not be psychologically ready for surgery or those who may not benefit from the procedure.

The psychological aspect of plastic surgery cannot be underestimated. Patients seeking cosmetic or reconstructive procedures often bring complex emotional and psychological factors to the decision-making process. Plastic surgeons must approach each case with sensitivity, empathy, and a focus on patient well-being. By addressing the psychological aspect alongside the physical, plastic surgery can be a transformative and rewarding experience for patients, enhancing their lives beyond the surface.

Chapter 5: The Surgeon-Patient Relationship

The surgeon-patient relationship is a fundamental aspect of plastic surgery that greatly influences the overall experience and outcomes for both parties. This unique bond is built on trust, communication, and empathy, creating a partnership that is essential for successful surgical journeys. Let's explore the key elements that contribute to a positive and productive surgeon-patient relationship:

1. Open and Honest Communication: Effective communication is the cornerstone of any successful relationship, and the surgeon-patient dynamic is no exception. A skilled plastic surgeon listens actively to the patient's concerns, desires, and goals. Patients, in turn, must be open and honest about their expectations, medical history, and any fears or anxieties they may have about the procedure.

2. Establishing Trust and Rapport:
Building trust is a vital component of the surgeon-patient relationship. Trust is established through the surgeon's expertise, experience, and commitment to patient well-being. Patients should feel comfortable discussing their concerns, knowing that their surgeon has their best interests at heart.

3. Informed Consent:
Informed consent is a critical aspect of the surgeon-patient relationship. It involves the surgeon providing comprehensive information about the procedure, potential risks, benefits, and expected outcomes. Patients must fully understand the implications of the surgery and voluntarily consent to proceed.

4. Realistic Expectations:
A key responsibility of the plastic surgeon is to set realistic expectations with the patient. Patients must understand what can and cannot be achieved through surgery. A skilled surgeon will ensure that the patient has a

clear understanding of the potential results, keeping their expectations in line with the procedure's limitations.

5. Individualized Treatment Plans:
Each patient is unique, and a successful surgeon-patient relationship involves tailoring the treatment plan to meet individual needs. A personalized approach takes into account the patient's medical history, anatomy, lifestyle, and aesthetic goals.

6. Emotional Support and Empathy:
Plastic surgery can be an emotionally significant experience for patients. Surgeons must approach the process with empathy and provide emotional support throughout the journey. This support includes addressing anxieties, managing expectations, and ensuring patients feel cared for and valued.

7. Post-Surgical Care and Follow-up:
The surgeon-patient relationship extends beyond the operating room. Follow-up care is essential to monitor recovery, address any concerns, and ensure patients are healing

well. Continuing communication and support during the post-operative period contribute to successful outcomes and patient satisfaction.

8. Safety and Ethical Considerations: Surgeons have a duty to prioritize patient safety and ethical considerations. This involves providing honest assessments of the risks and benefits of the procedure, adhering to medical guidelines, and turning away patients who may not be suitable candidates for surgery.

The surgeon-patient relationship is a dynamic partnership built on trust, communication, and mutual respect. Effective communication, empathy, and personalized care are essential for creating a positive and supportive environment for patients seeking plastic surgery. By fostering a strong surgeon-patient relationship, plastic surgeons can enhance patient satisfaction, optimize outcomes, and contribute to the overall well-being and confidence of their patients.

Chapter 6: Plastic Surgery and Self-Esteem

Plastic surgery can have a significant impact on self-esteem for many patients. While the relationship between plastic surgery and self-esteem is complex and varies among individuals, certain factors contribute to the positive influence plastic surgery can have on one's self-esteem:

1. Addressing Physical Insecurities: Plastic surgery can address specific physical features or imperfections that patients may be self-conscious about. Correcting these insecurities can lead to increased self-confidence and improved body image.

2. Feeling Empowered: Choosing to undergo plastic surgery is often a proactive decision, and taking control of one's appearance can empower individuals to feel more confident and satisfied with themselves.

3. Psychological Benefits: Research has shown that some patients experience psychological benefits after successful plastic surgery, such as improved self-esteem, reduced social anxiety, and a more positive self-perception.

4. Enhanced Self-Perception: Positive changes to one's appearance through plastic surgery can lead to a more favorable self-

perception. Feeling more attractive and content with one's looks can positively impact various aspects of life, including social interactions and career opportunities.

5. Overcoming Body Dysmorphia: In some cases, plastic surgery can help individuals with Body Dysmorphic Disorder (BDD) by correcting perceived flaws and alleviating distress associated with their appearance.

It is essential to note that plastic surgery is not a universal solution for all self-esteem issues. While some patients experience a boost in self-confidence and well-being, others may not achieve the same results or may experience temporary improvements.

Patients considering plastic surgery should have realistic expectations about the procedure's potential impact on their self-esteem and overall happiness. It is essential for individuals to undergo pre-surgical counseling and to choose reputable plastic surgeons who prioritize patient well-being and ethical considerations.

Ultimately, plastic surgery's impact on self-esteem varies, and success depends on multiple factors, including the patient's motivation, emotional well-being, and the surgeon's ability to provide a comprehensive assessment and tailored treatment plan. A balanced approach to plastic surgery, combined with an emphasis on personal growth and self-acceptance, can lead to the most positive and fulfilling outcomes for patients seeking to enhance their self-esteem through surgical means.

Chapter 7: Navigating the Risks and Complications

Navigating the risks and complications associated with plastic surgery is a crucial aspect of the decision-making process for both patients and surgeons. While plastic surgery is generally safe, like any medical procedure, it carries inherent risks. Understanding these potential risks and taking necessary precautions can help minimize complications and ensure a safer surgical experience. Here are some important considerations:

1. Pre-Surgical Evaluation:
Thorough pre-surgical evaluations are essential to identify any underlying health conditions or risk factors that may increase the likelihood of complications during or after surgery. Patients must disclose their complete medical history and any medications they are taking to the surgeon.

2. Surgeon Qualifications and Experience:
Choosing a qualified and experienced plastic surgeon is crucial to reduce the risk of complications. Research the surgeon's credentials, board certifications, and experience in performing the specific procedure you are considering.

3. Informed Consent:
Informed consent is a vital step in the surgical process, where the surgeon explains the risks, benefits, and potential complications associated with the procedure. Patients must fully understand the information provided before consenting to the surgery.

4. Anesthesia Risks:
Anesthesia carries its own set of risks, and patients should be aware of potential side effects or complications associated with the type of anesthesia used. Qualified anesthesiologists or certified nurse anesthetists should administer anesthesia.

5. Bleeding and Infection:
Bleeding and infection are potential risks associated with any surgical procedure. Proper post-operative care and adherence to the surgeon's instructions can help reduce these risks.

6. Scarring and Wound Healing:
While plastic surgeons aim to minimize scarring, some degree of scarring is inevitable

with surgery. Wound healing can vary from patient to patient, and factors such as genetics and following post-operative care instructions can influence the outcome.

7. Nerve Damage and Sensation Changes:
Certain procedures, especially those involving the face, can carry a risk of temporary or permanent nerve damage, leading to altered sensation or numbness in the operated area.

8. Unsatisfactory Results:
Plastic surgery outcomes can be influenced by several factors, including individual healing and patient expectations. Patients must have realistic expectations and understand that results may not be perfect or immediate.

9. Hematoma and Seroma:
Hematoma refers to the accumulation of blood under the skin, while seroma is a buildup of fluid. Both can occur after surgery and may require drainage to prevent complications.

10. Deep Vein Thrombosis (DVT) and Pulmonary Embolism (PE):
Certain procedures, especially those involving long periods of immobility, may increase the risk of DVT and PE, which are serious conditions. Patients should follow post-operative mobility guidelines and take preventive measures.

11. Allergic Reactions:
Patients must inform their surgeon about any known allergies to prevent potential allergic reactions to medications or materials used during surgery.

While plastic surgery can yield transformative results, it is essential to understand and navigate the associated risks and complications. A thorough evaluation, honest communication with the surgeon, and adherence to pre and post-operative instructions can significantly reduce risks and ensure a safer surgical experience. Patients should have a realistic understanding of the potential outcomes and be prepared for the recovery process to achieve the most satisfying results from their plastic surgery journey.

Chapter 8: Embracing Natural Beauty

Embracing natural beauty is an empowering and liberating mindset that celebrates individuality, self-acceptance, and authenticity. It encourages us to recognize and cherish our unique features, both physical and non-physical, rather than striving for an idealized or homogenized standard of beauty.

Here are some key aspects of embracing natural beauty:

1. Self-Acceptance:
Embracing natural beauty begins with accepting and appreciating ourselves as we are. It involves acknowledging that each person is inherently valuable and worthy, regardless of their appearance or perceived flaws.

2. Rejecting Unrealistic Beauty Standards:
Society often imposes unrealistic and narrow beauty standards, perpetuated by media and social platforms. Embracing natural beauty involves challenging these notions and recognizing that beauty comes in diverse forms.

3. Understanding the Impact of Social Media:
Social media can heavily influence perceptions of beauty and self-worth. It's essential to recognize that the images and portrayals we encounter online are often edited and curated, not reflective of reality.

4. Encouraging Individuality:
Natural beauty celebrates individuality and encourages people to express themselves authentically. Embracing our unique qualities fosters a sense of confidence and empowerment.

5. Redefining Beauty:
Embracing natural beauty involves redefining what beauty means to us personally. It's about recognizing that beauty is not confined to physical appearance but encompasses qualities like kindness, compassion, and inner strength.

6. Nurturing Physical and Mental Well-being:
Prioritizing self-care and overall well-being helps cultivate a positive self-image. Engaging in activities that make us feel good, such as exercise, healthy eating, and spending time in nature, can boost self-esteem and body positivity.

7. Supporting Others:

Promoting natural beauty also involves supporting others in their journey towards self-acceptance. Encouraging friends, family, and community members to embrace their natural beauty creates a positive and inclusive environment.

8. Mindful Consumption of Media:
Being mindful of the media we consume and the messages it conveys about beauty is crucial. Limiting exposure to harmful or unrealistic portrayals can protect our mental well-being and promote a more positive self-image.

9. Celebrating Aging:
Embracing natural beauty at any age includes celebrating the aging process as a natural part of life. Aging is a reflection of our experiences and wisdom, and it should be embraced with pride and grace.

10. Gratitude for the Body:
Developing a sense of gratitude for our bodies and all they do for us fosters a positive relationship with ourselves. Appreciating our

bodies for their strength and resilience enhances self-compassion.

Embracing natural beauty is an ongoing journey of self-discovery, self-acceptance, and self-love. It's about recognizing that we are all uniquely beautiful and deserving of love and respect just as we are. By embracing natural beauty and celebrating individuality, we contribute to a more inclusive and compassionate society, where everyone feels valued and accepted for their authentic selves.

Chapter 9: Ethical and Cultural Considerations

Ethical and cultural considerations play a vital role in the practice of plastic surgery, ensuring that patient care is respectful, sensitive, and aligned with ethical principles. These considerations extend beyond medical expertise and technical skills, emphasizing the importance of understanding and respecting diverse cultural beliefs, values, and social norms. Here are some key ethical and cultural considerations in plastic surgery:

1. Informed Consent:

Respecting a patient's autonomy and right to make informed decisions is paramount. Surgeons must provide comprehensive information about the procedure, including potential risks, benefits, and alternatives. This ensures that patients fully understand the implications of the surgery before giving their informed consent.

2. Cultural Sensitivity:
Cultural sensitivity involves recognizing and understanding cultural differences and adapting care accordingly. Surgeons should be attentive to cultural norms, beliefs, and practices that may impact a patient's decision to undergo plastic surgery or their expectations of the outcome.

3. Body Image and Beauty Standards:
Plastic surgeons must be mindful of the influence of cultural beauty standards on patient desires for specific procedures. Unrealistic or imposed beauty ideals can contribute to body dysmorphia and dissatisfaction. Encouraging patients to have

realistic expectations and promoting a diverse range of beauty standards is essential.

4. Gender-Affirming Surgery:
Gender-affirming surgery requires a deep understanding of the unique needs and experiences of transgender and gender-nonconforming patients. Plastic surgeons should provide gender-affirming care in a respectful, supportive, and affirming manner.

5. Ethical Marketing and Advertising:
Plastic surgeons should uphold ethical standards when marketing their services. Avoiding deceptive practices or unrealistic promises helps protect patients from making uninformed decisions based on advertising alone.

6. Patient Safety:
Ensuring patient safety is a fundamental ethical responsibility. Surgeons should thoroughly assess patients' medical history, fitness for surgery, and potential risks. They must prioritize patient well-being over financial interests.

7. Resource Allocation:
In regions with limited healthcare resources, ethical considerations may arise in allocating plastic surgery services. Balancing aesthetic procedures with reconstructive surgeries for medical need can be ethically challenging.

8. Cultural Competency Training:
Healthcare professionals, including plastic surgeons, should undergo cultural competency training to enhance their understanding of diverse cultural backgrounds and improve patient care.

9. Respect for Religious Beliefs:
Respecting patients' religious beliefs is essential. Some religious practices may impact a patient's readiness for surgery or post-operative care, and surgeons should be mindful and accommodating.

10. Respect for Modesty and Privacy:
Some cultures prioritize modesty and privacy. Surgeons should be sensitive to cultural preferences for attire, gender-specific care,

and privacy during examinations and consultations.

Ethical and cultural considerations are integral to the practice of plastic surgery. Emphasizing patient autonomy, cultural sensitivity, and respect for diverse beliefs and values contributes to patient-centered care and enhances the overall patient experience. By fostering a culture of ethical awareness and cultural competency, plastic surgeons can promote inclusivity, trust, and positive outcomes for their patients across diverse communities and backgrounds.

Chapter 10: Reconstructive Surgery and Humanitarian Efforts

Reconstructive surgery and humanitarian efforts intersect in powerful ways, offering life-changing transformations to individuals who have faced trauma, congenital deformities, or injuries in regions affected by conflict or limited access to medical care. These efforts go beyond cosmetic enhancements, aiming to restore function, dignity, and hope to those in need. Here are some key aspects of reconstructive surgery and humanitarian efforts:

1. Restoring Function and Quality of Life: Reconstructive surgery focuses on restoring function and form to body parts that have been affected by congenital conditions, accidents, burns, or disease. It aims to improve mobility, alleviate pain, and enhance overall quality of life for patients.

2. Addressing Cleft Lip and Palate:
Cleft lip and palate repair is a significant part of humanitarian reconstructive surgery. Correcting these congenital conditions helps children eat, speak, and breathe more effectively, enabling them to lead healthier lives.

3. Reconstructive Surgeries in Conflict Zones:
In regions affected by conflict, reconstructive surgery becomes a vital humanitarian effort. Surgeons provide life-changing interventions for individuals who have experienced devastating injuries, including facial trauma and limb amputations.

4. Non-Governmental Organizations (NGOs):
Numerous NGOs, medical missions, and volunteer organizations focus on providing reconstructive surgery to underserved populations. These efforts often involve collaborative partnerships between medical professionals and local communities.

5. Training Local Healthcare Providers:
Humanitarian efforts often include training local healthcare providers in reconstructive surgery techniques. This capacity-building approach helps create sustainable, long-term solutions to address the medical needs of the community.

6. Craniofacial Surgeries:
Craniofacial surgeries are crucial in humanitarian efforts, especially for children with complex craniofacial deformities. These surgeries not only improve physical function but also alleviate social stigmatization and enhance overall well-being.

7. Treating Burns and Trauma:
Reconstructive surgery plays a significant role in treating burn injuries and trauma victims. Restoring damaged tissue and providing scar revision can improve function, mobility, and appearance.

8. Collaborations with Local Communities:
Successful humanitarian reconstructive surgery initiatives involve collaborating

closely with local communities and respecting their cultural norms and beliefs. Engaging community leaders and understanding their healthcare needs is vital for successful outcomes.

9. Prosthetic and Orthotic Services:
Humanitarian efforts may also include providing prosthetic limbs or orthotic devices to individuals who have experienced limb amputations or musculoskeletal injuries, enabling them to regain mobility and independence.

10. Psychological Support:
In addition to surgical interventions, humanitarian efforts often incorporate psychological support and counseling for patients and their families. Addressing the emotional trauma associated with injuries and deformities is integral to the healing process.

Reconstructive surgery and humanitarian efforts are a testament to the power of compassion and medical expertise. They offer hope, healing, and renewed possibilities to individuals facing physical challenges in regions with limited access to healthcare. By combining surgical skills, cultural sensitivity, and collaborative partnerships, these efforts empower communities and transform lives, proving that the impact of medicine can extend far beyond borders and touch the hearts of those in need.

CONCLUSION

In conclusion, plastic surgery is a multifaceted discipline that touches on various aspects of human life. From its ancient origins to modern advancements, plastic surgery has evolved into a diverse field encompassing cosmetic enhancements, reconstructive procedures, and transformative surgeries that go beyond physical appearance. This book has explored the world of plastic surgery, shedding light on its history, types of procedures, and the profound impact it can have on individuals' lives.

Traveling on a budget is an art that demands resourcefulness, creativity, and a spirit of adventure. This book has provided a comprehensive guide, offering tips and tricks to help travelers explore the world without breaking the bank. From planning a budget adventure and saving on transportation and accommodation to savoring budget-friendly cuisine and engaging in savvy sightseeing, the pages of this book have been a roadmap to an enriching and affordable travel experience.

Furthermore, this book has delved into the psychological aspect of plastic surgery, emphasizing the importance of understanding patients' motivations and promoting self-acceptance and realistic expectations. By addressing the emotional journey alongside the physical transformation, plastic surgery can be a catalyst for positive change and enhanced well-being.

Ethical and cultural considerations are integral to the practice of plastic surgery and play a crucial role in ensuring patient-centered care. By embracing natural beauty and celebrating individuality, plastic surgeons can foster a positive surgeon-patient relationship and promote a diverse and inclusive approach to beauty.

Lastly, the book has highlighted the altruistic side of plastic surgery through humanitarian efforts. Reconstructive surgery serves as a beacon of hope, restoring function and dignity to those in need, often in regions affected by conflict or limited access to medical care. By engaging in collaborations with local communities and embracing a spirit of compassion, humanitarian reconstructive surgery transforms lives and spreads healing across borders.

As we close this book, let us remember that both plastic surgery and budget travel are journeys that involve growth, self-discovery, and empowerment. They exemplify the boundless potential of human endeavor, demonstrating that with knowledge, compassion, and a sense of purpose, we can make a positive impact on ourselves and the world around us.

May the wisdom shared in this book inspire readers to explore the depths of their own possibilities, make informed choices, and embrace the beauty of life, wherever it may lead. As we venture forth, let us remember that the journey is as valuable as the destination, and that the true essence of traveling on a budget and plastic surgery lies in making memories, embracing authenticity, and navigating life's challenges with resilience and grace.